East Asian Diet

A Beginner's Step-by-Step Guide with Recipes and a Meal Plan

mf

copyright © 2022 Bruce Ackerberg

All rights reserved No part of this book may be reproduced, or stored in a retrieval system, or transmitted in any form or by any means, electronic, mechanical, photocopying, recording, or otherwise, without express written permission of the publisher.

Disclaimer

By reading this disclaimer, you are accepting the terms of the disclaimer in full. If you disagree with this disclaimer, please do not read the guide.

All of the content within this guide is provided for informational and educational purposes only, and should not be accepted as independent medical or other professional advice. The author is not a doctor, physician, nurse, mental health provider, or registered nutritionist/dietician. Therefore, using and reading this guide does not establish any form of a physician-patient relationship.

Always consult with a physician or another qualified health provider with any issues or questions you might have regarding any sort of medical condition. Do not ever disregard any qualified professional medical advice or delay seeking that advice because of anything you have read in this guide. The information in this guide is not intended to be any sort of medical advice and should not be used in lieu of any medical advice by a licensed and qualified medical professional.

The information in this guide has been compiled from a variety of known sources. However, the author cannot attest to or guarantee the accuracy of each source and thus should not be held liable for any errors or omissions.

You acknowledge that the publisher of this guide will not be held liable for any loss or damage of any kind incurred as a result of this guide or the reliance on any information provided within this guide. You acknowledge and agree that you assume all risk and responsibility for any action you undertake in response to the information in this guide.

Using this guide does not guarantee any particular result (e.g., weight loss or a cure). By reading this guide, you acknowledge that there are no guarantees to any specific outcome or results you can expect.

All product names, diet plans, or names used in this guide are for identification purposes only and are the property of their respective owners. The use of these names does not imply endorsement. All other trademarks cited herein are the property of their respective owners.

Where applicable, this guide is not intended to be a substitute for the original work of this diet plan and is, at most, a supplement to the original work for this diet plan and never a direct substitute. This guide is a personal expression of the facts of that diet plan.

Where applicable, persons shown in the cover images are stock photography models and the publisher has obtained the rights to use the images through license agreements with third-party stock image companies.

Table of Contents

Introduction	7
What Is the East Asian Diet?	10
Principles of the East Asian Diet	11
The Benefits of the East Asian Diet	13
Disadvantages of the East Asian Diet	15
Use Cases of East Asian Diet	18
How Does the Diet Work?	20
Important Points of the East Asian Diet to Remember	22
5 Step-by-Step Guide on How to Get Started with The East Asian Diet	25
Step 1: Fill Your Plate with Vegetables	25
Step 2: Incorporate Whole Grains	28
Step 3: Choose Lean Proteins	31
Step 4: Savor Fruits as Snacks or Desserts	34
Step 5: Experiment with Fermented Foods	37
Foods Included in the East Asian Diet Plan	39
Foods to Avoid	41
Sample 7-Day Meal Plan	43
Sample Recipes	47
Roasted Chicken Banh Mi	48
Chicken Thigh Hoisin-Style with Salad	50
Miso Vegetable Soup Recipe	52
Shrimp Fried Rice	54
Ginger Beef Stir-Fry with Bok Choy	56
Spinach Salad Mixed with Ginger Dressing	58
Cantonese-Style Vegetable and Chicken Combo	60
Kimchi Fried Rice	62
Chinese Noodle Salad with Sesame Dressing	64
Peanut Butter Noodles	66

Korean-Style Seasoned Spinach (Sigeumchi Namul)	68
Fresh Spring Rolls with Peanut Dipping Sauce	69
Mixed Berry Smoothie Bowl	71
Broccoli with Cashews and Garlic Butter	72
Fish Congee	73
Chicken & Green Pepper Stir Fry	75
Cantonese Shiu Mai Dumplings	77
Conclusion	**79**
FAQ	**82**
References and Helpful Links	**84**

Introduction

In an era where the pursuit of health often leads us through a maze of fleeting diet trends and short-lived exercise fads, the East Asian diet emerges as a testament to the enduring value of tradition and equilibrium. This guide offers a gentle introduction to a dietary practice that has sustained generations, highlighting the importance of whole foods, diverse selections, and the joy found in shared meals. It opens a door to a lifestyle that prizes harmony with the natural world and thoughtful consumption, promising a positive impact on overall well-being.

The charm of the East Asian diet resides in its straightforward yet profound approach. This culinary heritage, abundant in vegetables, fruits, whole grains, and lean proteins, provides a well-rounded selection from which tasty and healthful meals are crafted. The diet promotes a respectful and grateful relationship with food, encouraging a way of eating that is as beneficial as it is pleasurable. Each meal is a chance to appreciate the taste of unprocessed ingredients, thoughtfully prepared and served to enhance their healthful properties and flavors.

For those curious about incorporating these values into their own dietary habits, this guide shines a light on the path forward. It advocates for adopting eating practices that not only support personal health but also consider environmental sustainability. The East Asian diet isn't about making dramatic changes or sticking strictly to rules. Rather, it recommends mindful decisions and gradual adjustments that can foster better health, increased vitality, and greater contentment with one's dietary choices.

In this guide, we will talk about the following;

- What is the East Asian Diet?
- Use Cases of East Asian Diet
- How Does the Diet Work?
- Important Points of the East Asian Diet to Remember
- 5 Step-by-Step Guide on How to Get Started with The East Asian Diet
- Foods to Eat and To Avoid
- 7-Day Sample Meal Plan and Recipes

This guide marks the beginning of your exploration into how the East Asian diet can seamlessly integrate into your daily life. With practical advice, easy-to-follow recipes, and insights into the cultural significance of various foods and customs, you'll discover how to make choices that resonate with a balanced and healthy approach to eating. Whether you're an avid food lover aiming to broaden your culinary horizons or someone seeking a sustainable method to enhance your diet, this introduction offers a rewarding experience that is both enriching and appetizing.

We invite you to delve into the principles, customs, and delights of the East Asian diet. More than just providing recipes, this guide introduces a fresh viewpoint on nutrition and health, shaped by centuries of insight. It extends an invitation to engage in the art of balanced eating—a voyage that enriches the body satisfies the senses and elevates the spirit.

What Is the East Asian Diet?

The East Asian Diet, which encompasses the culinary cultures of many countries in the Asian continent, is a time-honored and ancient way of eating. For millennia, Asians have eaten a plant-based diet consisting mostly of vegetables, rice, and fruit. As compared to Western diets, the East Asian Diet uses meat as a supplement, not as the main course. The exception is fish, which is consumed daily.

The East Asian Diet is linked closely to tradition and religious practices. Asians who have access to various traditional, fresh foods are some of the world's wealthiest individuals. Chronic illnesses that affect the West like cancer, heart disease, and obesity are relatively rare in East Asian cultures.

In the East Asian Diet, religious and philosophical practices mostly dictate the kinds of food consumed. Moreover, mealtimes are vital for family relationships. The East Asian Diet is based on fresh food that is steamed, left raw, deep-fried, or stir-fried.

The East Asian Diet is influenced by agriculture, religion, and culture. High in fiber, low in fat, and full of fresh vegetables and fruit, many believe that the East Asian Diet is the secret to a healthy and lengthy life. When you eat a plant-based diet, you tend to eat fewer calories. The way of cooking and the spices stimulate the palate and help you feel full and satisfied.

Principles of the East Asian Diet

The East Asian diet is rooted in principles that have evolved over millennia, reflecting a deep understanding of nutrition and its effects on health according to traditional practices and modern interpretations. These principles include:

1. ***Balance and Moderation***: At the core of the East Asian diet is the idea of maintaining balance and moderation in all things, including food. This principle is about consuming a variety of foods without overindulgence in any specific type or nutrient.
2. ***Whole and Minimally Processed Foods***: Emphasis is placed on eating foods that are as close to their natural state as possible. This includes whole grains, fresh vegetables and fruits, and minimally processed proteins like fish and legumes.
3. ***Dietary Diversity***: The diet advocates for a wide range of foods to ensure nutritional completeness. This diversity also reflects the traditional agricultural practices and regional variations across East Asia.

4. ***Plant-Based Focus***: While not exclusively vegetarian, the East Asian diet leans heavily towards plant-based foods, with meat and animal products often used sparingly and as flavor enhancers rather than centerpieces of a meal.
5. ***Inclusion of Fermented Foods***: Fermented foods such as kimchi, miso, and fermented tofu play a significant role in the diet, contributing to gut health and providing a unique set of nutrients and probiotics.
6. ***Mindful Eating***: The practice of eating mindfully and with gratitude is emphasized, encouraging individuals to pay attention to the flavors, textures, and nutritional value of their food, as well as to eat at a slower pace.
7. ***Seasonal and Local Eating***: There is a strong emphasis on consuming foods that are in season and locally sourced, aligning with the natural cycles and reducing the environmental impact of food consumption.
8. ***Therapeutic Use of Foods***: Foods are considered for their therapeutic properties, with certain diets tailored to address specific health concerns or to promote overall well-being according to the principles of traditional Chinese medicine.
9. ***Five Flavors Balance***: The diet incorporates the traditional concept of balancing the five key flavors—sweet, sour, salty, bitter, and umami. This not

only ensures a pleasurable eating experience but is also believed to contribute to internal balance and health.
10. *Cooking Methods*: Preference is given to cooking methods that preserve the integrity and nutritional value of ingredients, such as steaming, boiling, and quick stir-frying, over high-fat or high-heat methods.

These principles together form a holistic approach to eating that is geared towards nourishing the body, promoting longevity, and maintaining a harmonious balance between the individual and the natural world.

The Benefits of the East Asian Diet

Certainly, focusing purely on the benefits that are distinct from the specific disease management use cases previously mentioned, the East Asian diet offers a broad spectrum of general health advantages:

- *Enhanced Digestive Health*: Beyond just gut flora balance, the high fiber content improves overall digestive function, reducing the risk of constipation and promoting regular bowel movements.
- *Improved Skin Health*: The antioxidants and omega-3 fatty acids prevalent in the diet can contribute to healthier skin, potentially reducing signs of aging and decreasing the prevalence of acne and other skin conditions.

- *Increased Energy Levels*: Balanced macronutrient distribution ensures a steady supply of energy throughout the day, preventing the spikes and crashes associated with diets high in refined sugars.
- *Strengthened Immune System*: A variety of vitamins and minerals, particularly those found in the colorful fruits and vegetables of the East Asian diet, support a robust immune system, helping the body fend off illnesses.
- *Better Hydration*: Traditional East Asian diets emphasize soups and broths, which contribute to better hydration and can aid in maintaining electrolyte balance.
- *Enhanced Cognitive Function*: Nutrients like omega-3 fatty acids, flavonoids, and antioxidants may improve focus, memory, and overall brain health, potentially reducing the risk of cognitive decline with age.
- *Mood Regulation*: The diet's emphasis on whole foods and balanced nutrition can have a positive impact on mood, contributing to reduced stress levels and a lower risk of depression.
- *Improved Sleep Quality*: Certain elements of the East Asian diet, such as magnesium-rich foods and those that promote serotonin production, may contribute to better sleep patterns and quality.

- ***Lowered Blood Pressure***: The combination of low sodium intake and high potassium intake from fruits, vegetables, and legumes can contribute to lower blood pressure levels.
- ***Sustainable Weight Loss***: The emphasis on whole foods and natural ingredients helps promote satiety and control hunger, supporting sustainable weight loss and maintenance without drastic calorie restriction.

These benefits underscore the holistic impact of the East Asian diet on overall well-being, highlighting its role not just in disease prevention and management, but also in promoting a vibrant, healthy lifestyle.

Disadvantages of the East Asian Diet

While the East Asian diet offers a plethora of health benefits, like any dietary approach, it may come with certain disadvantages or challenges for some individuals. However, it's important to note that for many, the benefits significantly outweigh these potential drawbacks. Here are some considerations:

- ***Cultural and Palatability Adjustments***: Individuals not accustomed to East Asian flavors and cooking styles may find it challenging to adapt to this diet, potentially limiting their enjoyment and long-term adherence.

- *Soy Allergies and Sensitivities*: The diet's reliance on soy products as a primary protein source can pose problems for those with soy allergies or sensitivities, requiring careful substitution planning.
- *Seafood Contaminants*: Given the prominence of fish and seafood, there's a risk of exposure to contaminants like mercury and microplastics, especially if not carefully sourced.
- *Limited Access to Authentic Ingredients*: Depending on one's location, accessing fresh, authentic East Asian ingredients can be difficult and potentially more expensive, which might discourage some individuals.
- *Preparation Time*: Traditional East Asian meals can sometimes require extensive preparation time, which may not fit into everyone's busy lifestyles, leading to a preference for quicker, less nutritious options.
- *Potential for Imbalance*: Without proper knowledge or guidance, there's a risk of nutritional imbalances, such as inadequate calcium or iron intake, especially among those who may not diversify their food choices within the diet's framework.
- *Rice-Heavy Meals*: A traditional emphasis on white rice can lead to excessive carbohydrate intake for some individuals, particularly if portion sizes are not managed or if there's insufficient incorporation of whole grains.

Despite these potential disadvantages, the East Asian diet remains highly beneficial for many, primarily due to its focus on whole, minimally processed foods, diversity of plant-based ingredients, lean proteins, and healthy fats.

When approached with mindfulness and adaptations to meet individual nutritional needs and preferences, the East Asian diet can significantly contribute to improved health outcomes, including better heart health, weight management, digestive health, and reduced risk of chronic diseases. The key is finding a balance and making informed choices that align with one's health goals while navigating any dietary limitations or concerns.

Use Cases of East Asian Diet

The East Asian diet, with its emphasis on whole, minimally processed foods, plant-based ingredients, and lean proteins, has been recognized for its potential to manage and potentially prevent various health conditions. Based on the context provided by recent findings and reports, here are several use cases or diseases that the East Asian diet can help to manage:

1. *Type 2 Diabetes Management*: The diet's low glycemic index foods and high fiber content can aid in blood sugar regulation, making it beneficial for individuals managing type 2 diabetes. The cultural considerations in dietary self-management for East Asian Americans also highlight the importance of tailoring diabetes care to accommodate traditional dietary preferences.
2. *Heart Disease Prevention*: By focusing on heart-healthy fats and a wide range of fruits and vegetables, the East Asian diet can lower the risk of heart disease. Reports suggest fine-tuning Asian diets

could further reduce the distinct risks of heart disease prevalent in these populations.
3. *Atherosclerotic Cardiovascular Disease (ASCVD)*: Nutritional management, including diets similar to the East Asian diet, has shown promise in decreasing the risk of ASCVD by emphasizing whole grains, lean proteins, and a variety of plant-based foods.
4. *Cancer Risk Reduction*: The inclusion of soybean-based foods and other plant-based foods rich in phytochemicals may contribute to a lower risk of certain cancers, including breast and prostate cancer, by offering protective effects against cellular damage.
5. *Nutritional Deficiencies*: The diverse and nutrient-rich nature of the East Asian diet helps combat nutritional deficiencies, contributing to overall health and well-being, especially in regions where suboptimal diets are a significant risk factor for disease.
6. *Chronic Kidney Disease*: For individuals with diabetes, the East Asian diet may help manage blood sugar levels and thus reduce the risk of complications such as chronic kidney disease, which is a common comorbidity.
7. *Noncommunicable Diseases (NCDs)*: Healthy food systems, like those promoted by the East Asian diet, can play a critical role in preventing NCDs by addressing their root causes related to diet and lifestyle.

8. ***Eating Disorders***: While the rise of eating disorders in Asia points to a global health challenge, integrating traditional dietary practices and principles can contribute to healthier eating patterns and attitudes toward food.
9. ***Stroke and Ischemic Heart Disease***: Given the mixed progress in combating health challenges in the East Asia and Pacific Region, adopting dietary patterns focused on reducing saturated fat intake and increasing consumption of fruits, vegetables, and whole grains could help address the rising incidence of stroke and ischemic heart disease.

By embracing the principles and foods characteristic of the East Asian diet, individuals may find effective strategies for managing these conditions, contributing to improved health outcomes and quality of life.

How Does the Diet Work?

The East Asian diet, characterized by its emphasis on whole foods and balance, operates in harmony with the body to promote health and well-being. At its core, this diet includes a generous consumption of vegetables, fruits, whole grains, soy products, and lean proteins such as fish, which are minimally processed. This combination ensures a high intake of dietary fiber, antioxidants, and essential nutrients, while maintaining low levels of saturated fats.

In the body, the fiber from whole grains and vegetables aids in digestion and helps maintain a healthy gut microbiome, crucial for optimal nutrient absorption and immune function. Antioxidants and nutrients from fruits and vegetables work to neutralize free radicals, reducing inflammation and lowering the risk of chronic diseases. The lean proteins and soy products provide essential amino acids for muscle repair and growth, without the added burden of unhealthy fats.

Overall, the East Asian diet supports cardiovascular health, aids in weight management, and contributes to a lower risk of metabolic diseases by fostering a nutritional balance that aligns with the body's natural needs.

Important Points of the East Asian Diet to Remember

When you take away the philosophies that go together with adhering to the East Asian Diet, the core of the diet is simply to attain and maintain wellness. Weight loss may just be merely a good by-product of following the diet. As you continue to follow the East Asian Diet, you will notice an overall health improvement.

Some of the important dietary habits of the East Asian Diet include:

1. *Consuming soup.* Soup is nutrient-rich and easily makes you full. Even half a cup of soup is beneficial. Many East Asian soups are made with vegetable combinations and/or bones, so you're getting a lot of nutrients.

    Whether they are miso vegetable soup, or bone broth, soups are rich in minerals and vitamins and are absorbed easily. Moreover, a soup's warm temperature can improve digestion.

2. ***Limiting drinks, especially cold drinks during meals***. A common Western mealtime habit is having a glass of cold water or soda together with meals. Changing this habit can vastly improve digestion. Limit your intake of fluid, and you will curb the dilution of important digestive enzymes.

   Hot teas like green tea eating support enzymes activity and help in overall digestion as well. Drink your liquids 30 minutes after or before meals, not during meals.

3. ***Chopsticks and small plates***. To eat smaller portions, use small plates and small serving bowls. Chopsticks are also useful when you want to avoid shoveling food into your mouth. When you eat with chopsticks, especially if you're a beginner, your food consumption rate slows, signaling to your brain that you're full.

4. ***Eat a 3:1 vegetable-to-meat ratio***. Eat three times as many vegetables to accompany your meal. Some excellent East Asian vegetables include radicchio, radish, and bitter melon.

5. ***Rice combinations***. Combining rice like red, brown, black, or purple leads to a rice variety with more nutrients than brown or white rice alone. In Asia, rice is more of a supplement – not the main dish. Combining rice results in less starchy rice, which is low-calorie and is not easily converted into sugar.

6. *Seafood*. Most Asians include fish in their daily diet.
7. *Dessert is not mandatory*. You may want to wash down your meal with a sweet treat. However, if you want to be healthy while doing it, eating cake is not the way to go. Fruit, especially fresh fruit, is the go-to East Asian dessert.
8. *Healthier snacks*. Healthier East Asian snacks would put your American cookies and chips to shame. Many of the East Asian snacks are nutritionally dense like dried seeds and fruit, nuts, seaweed snacks, sunflower seeds, and pumpkin seeds.
9. *Avoid milk combining and cow's milk*. Most East Asian diets do not have cow's milk in them. Moreover, cow's milk also does not mix well with anything. Some cow's milk substitutes include coconut, almond, soy, or rice milk.
10. *Optimize seasonal food temperatures*. Food temperature should be considered. In hot weather, eat cooling food. In cold weather, eat warm food. Cold food and cold drinks like melons, cold salads, and celery are not consumed during winter.

During cold weather, hot meat stews and soups are desired, since the body needs them during the cold. For the summer, consume a watermelon or enjoy a cooling drink from cucumber and aloe. Eating the appropriate temperature food is vital to a healthy diet.

5 Step-by-Step Guide on How to Get Started with The East Asian Diet

Embarking on the journey of adopting the East Asian diet involves embracing a philosophy that prioritizes balance, variety, and mindfulness in eating. Here's a straightforward guide to begin integrating this healthful and flavorful diet into your lifestyle:

Step 1: Fill Your Plate with Vegetables

Embarking on the East Asian diet journey begins with a vibrant and colorful transformation of your plate, where vegetables are elevated from mere sides to the centerpiece of your dining experience. This shift not only enriches your meals with a spectrum of flavors and nutrients but also aligns you with a centuries-old tradition of eating that emphasizes health and harmony.

1. **Diversify Your Vegetable Selection**

   The first step is to broaden your vegetable horizons. East Asian cuisine celebrates a vast array of vegetables, each bringing its unique nutritional profile and taste. Leafy greens such as bok choy, spinach, and Chinese cabbage are staples, rich in vitamins A, C, and K, as well as minerals like iron and calcium.

   Root vegetables like radishes, sweet potatoes, and lotus roots offer dietary fiber and a range of antioxidants. Don't overlook the beauty of colorful vegetables—bell peppers, eggplants, and tomatoes—to boost your intake of vitamins and phytonutrients. The goal is to incorporate a rainbow of vegetables into your diet, ensuring a wide variety of essential nutrients.

2. **Master Various Preparation Methods**

   Keeping your vegetable dishes exciting involves getting creative with how you prepare them. Steaming is a gentle way to cook vegetables, preserving their natural crunch and nutritional content. It's ideal for broccoli, carrots, and green beans, yielding tender yet crisp results. Boiling can be used for sturdier vegetables like potatoes and yams, making them soft and easy to digest.

   However, the star method in East Asian cooking is stir-frying. This quick, high-heat cooking technique keeps vegetables somewhat crisp and vibrant while infusing them with flavors from garlic, ginger, and soy sauce. Stir-frying not only makes the vegetables deliciously appetizing but also ensures they retain most of their vitamins and minerals.

3. **Integrate Vegetables into Every Meal**

   To truly adopt the East Asian approach, aim to include vegetables in every meal. Start your day with a vegetable omelet or a side of sautéed greens. For lunch and dinner, ensure that at least half of your plate is filled with a variety of cooked and raw vegetables. Even snacks can be an opportunity to increase your vegetable intake—think crisp cucumber slices, carrot sticks, or lightly steamed edamame.

4. **Explore Traditional Dishes**

   Delve into the world of traditional East Asian dishes that spotlight vegetables. Dishes such as vegetable stir-fries, salads dressed with sesame oil and vinegar, and soups brimming with tofu and seaweed can inspire your meal planning. These dishes not only offer a way to enjoy vegetables in their myriad forms but also connect you with the rich culinary traditions of East Asia.

By making vegetables the focal point of your meals, you're not just adhering to the East Asian diet; you're embarking on a journey towards a more healthful, balanced, and vibrant way of eating. This fundamental shift towards prioritizing vegetables introduces a plethora of flavors and textures to your diet, making each meal an opportunity to nourish your body and delight your palate.

Step 2: Incorporate Whole Grains

Transitioning to whole grains is a pivotal step in adopting the East Asian diet, marking a shift towards more nutrient-dense and healthful eating habits. Refined grains, such as white rice and white bread, have been stripped of their most nutritious parts during processing, leaving them with fewer vitamins, minerals, and fibers. Whole grains, on the other hand, retain all their natural goodness, including the bran, germ, and endosperm, making them a powerhouse of nutrition.

1. **Understand the Benefits of Whole Grains**

    Whole grains are not just about adding variety to your diet; they bring a host of health benefits. The fiber content in whole grains plays a crucial role in maintaining healthy digestion, and preventing constipation, and may help in managing weight by keeping you feeling full for longer periods.

    Furthermore, these grains are sources of essential nutrients, including B vitamins, iron, folate, selenium, potassium, and magnesium. Regular consumption of whole grains has been linked to a lower risk of heart disease, diabetes, certain cancers, and other health conditions.

2. **Explore a Variety of Whole Grains**

   The world of whole grains goes beyond just brown rice and whole wheat. Quinoa, although technically a seed, is prepared and eaten like a grain and is known for its high protein content and all nine essential amino acids, making it an excellent choice for vegetarians and vegans.

   Barley is another versatile grain, offering a chewy texture and nutty flavor, perfect for soups and stews. Millet, with its mild flavor, can be a great addition to salads or served as a side dish. Each grain has its unique taste and texture, providing endless opportunities to diversify your meals.

3. **Introduce Whole Grains Gradually**

   If you're new to whole grains, it's important to introduce them into your diet gradually. This allows your digestive system to adjust to the increased fiber intake. Start by mixing whole grains with refined grains, such as using half white rice and half brown rice, gradually increasing the proportion of whole grains.

Experiment with one new whole grain at a time to discover what you enjoy most and to learn how each can be best prepared.

4. **Learn How to Cook Whole Grains**

   Cooking whole grains is not much different from cooking their refined counterparts, but it may require some adjustments. Most whole grains need to be rinsed thoroughly before cooking to remove any dust or debris.

   Cooking times can vary significantly from one grain to another, with some grains requiring soaking to shorten the cooking time and enhance digestibility. Exploring different cooking methods, such as boiling, simmering, and even using a rice cooker or pressure cooker, can yield delicious and healthful results.

5. **Incorporate Whole Grains into Every Meal**

   Make whole grains a staple in your diet by incorporating them into each meal. Start your day with oatmeal or whole-grain pancakes. Use quinoa or barley in your lunch salads. Serve a side of brown rice or millet with dinner. Even snacks can include whole grains, such as popcorn or whole-grain crackers.

   By making whole grains a central part of your diet, you're not only embracing a key aspect of the East

Asian dietary philosophy but also taking significant steps towards improving your overall health. The variety of textures and flavors that whole grains offer can make your meals more interesting and satisfying, turning the act of eating into a nourishing and enjoyable experience.

Step 3: Choose Lean Proteins

Adopting lean proteins into your diet is a transformative step towards aligning with the East Asian dietary philosophy, which values moderation, balance, and the healthful benefits of a varied diet.

Lean proteins, such as fish, tofu, legumes, and eggs, not only offer essential nutrients but also support a sustainable and balanced approach to eating.

1. **Understanding the Benefits of Lean Proteins**

    Lean proteins are pivotal for muscle repair, immune function, and overall health. They provide essential amino acids without the excess saturated fats found in higher-fat meats, contributing to heart health and weight management.

    Fish, rich in omega-3 fatty acids, supports brain health and cardiovascular wellness. Tofu and legumes, apart from being excellent protein sources, bring additional benefits like fiber, vitamins, and minerals. Eggs, versatile and nutrient-dense, offer high-quality protein along with vitamins D and B12.

2. **Incorporating More Fish in Your Diet**

   The East Asian diet often highlights fish as a primary protein source. Incorporating a variety of fish, from fatty types like salmon and mackerel to leaner options like cod and tilapia, ensures a range of nutrients, including omega-3 fatty acids.

   Explore different cooking methods, such as grilling for a smoky flavor, poaching to preserve tenderness, or stir-frying for a quick and flavorful meal. Including fish in your diet a few times a week can significantly contribute to a balanced nutritional intake.

3. **Exploring Plant-Based Proteins**

   Tofu and legumes are cornerstone ingredients in many East Asian dishes, celebrated not just for their protein content but also for their versatility in cooking. Tofu can absorb flavors from spices and sauces, making it an excellent addition to stir-fries, soups, and salads.

   Legumes, such as lentils, beans, and chickpeas, can be used in a variety of dishes, from stews to curries, offering both protein and fiber. Experimenting with these plant-based proteins can open up a world of culinary possibilities while contributing to a more sustainable diet.

4. **Utilizing Eggs for Protein**

   Eggs are another versatile and affordable source of high-quality protein. They can be prepared in numerous ways - boiled, scrambled, poached, or used in omelets and frittatas, incorporating vegetables for an even more nutritious meal. Including eggs in your diet provides not only protein but also essential vitamins and minerals, contributing to a well-rounded nutritional profile.

5. **Reducing Intake of Red and Processed Meats**

   To fully embrace the East Asian approach to diet, it's important to reduce the consumption of red and processed meats. These meats are often higher in saturated fat and calories, and their excessive consumption has been linked to various health issues, including heart disease and certain cancers. Shifting towards leaner proteins supports not only personal health but also environmental sustainability.

By choosing lean proteins and incorporating them into your diet through various cooking methods, you enrich your meals with essential nutrients while adhering to the principles of balance and moderation central to the East Asian diet. This step not only enhances your culinary repertoire but also supports a healthier, more balanced lifestyle.

Step 4: Savor Fruits as Snacks or Desserts

Transforming your approach to snacks and desserts by favoring fruits over sugary alternatives is a delightful way to follow the East Asian dietary philosophy. This practice not only healthfully caters to your sweet cravings but also enriches your diet with a plethora of nutrients, including vitamins, minerals, fibers, and antioxidants, essential for overall health and well-being.

1. **Reap the Nutritional Benefits of Fruits**

    Fruits are nature's treat, packed with an array of vitamins such as Vitamin C, which supports immune function, and Vitamin A, important for vision and skin health. They are also rich in antioxidants, compounds that fight free radicals, reducing oxidative stress and lowering the risk of chronic diseases.

    Moreover, the fiber content in fruits promotes digestive health and helps in maintaining a healthy weight by keeping you fuller for longer. By making fruits your primary choice for snacks and desserts, you're not just indulging in their sweetness but also benefiting from their nutritional abundance.

2. **Creative Ways to Enjoy Fruits**

   While eating fresh fruits whole is one of the simplest ways to enjoy them, there are numerous creative methods to incorporate more fruits into your diet. Preparing smoothies is an excellent way to combine various fruits, and even vegetables, into a delicious and nutritious drink.

   Fruit salads, mixed with a squeeze of lemon or a drizzle of honey, can serve as a refreshing snack or dessert. Experiment with grilling fruits like pineapples or peaches to unlock a different flavor profile. You can also freeze grapes or berries for a cool treat, especially during warmer months.

3. **Incorporate Fruits in Every Meal**

   Beyond snacks and desserts, fruits can be integrated into every meal. Add sliced bananas or berries to your morning cereal or oatmeal. Incorporate diced apples or oranges into salads for a burst of freshness. Use fruit purees as natural sweeteners in baking, reducing the need for added sugars. By making fruits a staple in your diet, you ensure a constant intake of essential nutrients throughout the day.

4. **Embrace Seasonal and Local Fruits**

   To fully enjoy the benefits and flavors of fruits, opt for seasonal and locally sourced options whenever possible. Seasonal fruits are picked at their peak of ripeness, ensuring the best taste and nutritional value.

Supporting local produce also contributes to sustainability and helps reduce your carbon footprint. Exploring farmers' markets can introduce you to a variety of regional fruits you might not find in conventional grocery stores, expanding your palate and culinary possibilities.

5. **Fruits as Digestive Aids**

The practice of consuming fruits before meals, valued in East Asian cultures, is based on the belief that certain fruits can aid digestion. Fruits like papaya, pineapple, and kiwi contain natural enzymes that help break down proteins, making them excellent pre-meal choices.

This practice not only prepares the digestive system for the upcoming meal but also ensures you start your meal with a nutrient-rich choice.

By making fruits the centerpiece of your snacks and desserts, you're not just healthily satisfying your sweet tooth; you're also embracing a lifestyle that values nutrition, variety, and the joy of eating. Fruits offer a delightful array of flavors and textures, making every bite a step towards a healthier, more balanced diet.

Step 5: Experiment with Fermented Foods

Incorporating fermented foods into your diet marks a significant stride towards embracing the full spectrum of the East Asian dietary philosophy. Fermented foods such as kimchi, miso, and tempeh are not only staples in East Asian cuisine but also offer profound health benefits, particularly for the digestive system.

These foods undergo a natural fermentation process where beneficial bacteria break down food components, resulting in the creation of probiotics, enzymes, and increased nutrient levels.

1. **Understanding the Probiotic Power**

    The primary allure of fermented foods lies in their rich probiotic content. Probiotics are beneficial bacteria that play an essential role in maintaining gut health, aiding digestion, and supporting the immune system.

    Regular consumption of fermented foods can help balance the gut microbiota, which is crucial for overall health. By introducing these foods into your diet, you're not just enhancing flavors but also fortifying your body's natural defenses.

2. **Starting with Small Portions**

    If you're new to fermented foods, it's wise to start with small amounts and gradually increase your intake. This approach allows your digestive system to adjust to the probiotics and prevents any potential discomfort.

A side of kimchi with your dinner, a spoonful of miso paste to enrich soups and marinades, or a slice of tempeh in your stir-fry are excellent ways to begin experimenting with these flavorful ingredients.

3. Diverse Ways to Enjoy Fermented Foods

Beyond their health benefits, fermented foods offer a unique depth of flavor to dishes. Kimchi, with its spicy and tangy profile, can be a vibrant addition to rice dishes, and stews, and even as a topping on burgers. Miso paste, with its salty and umami-rich taste, is incredibly versatile—perfect for seasoning soups, sauces, and dressings.

Tempeh, known for its nutty flavor and firm texture, can be marinated and grilled, making it an excellent protein source for vegetarians and meat-eaters alike. Experimenting with these foods can open up a new dimension of culinary possibilities, adding complexity and richness to your meals.

4. Incorporate Fermented Foods into Daily Meals

To fully reap the benefits of fermented foods, aim to include them in your daily diet. Breakfast could feature a miso soup, lunch could include a serving of tempeh salad, and dinner might be complemented with a side of kimchi. Even snacks can be an opportunity to enjoy fermented foods, such as yogurt or kefir, which are also rich in probiotics.

5. **Explore Making Your Own Fermented Foods**

   For those interested in a hands-on approach, consider preparing fermented foods at home. Fermenting vegetables like cabbage to make your own kimchi or cucumbers for pickles can be a rewarding experience.

Not only does this allow you to control the ingredients and level of fermentation, but it also connects you with traditional food preservation methods. Home fermentation is a journey of discovery, yielding delicious results that benefit your health and palate.

By following these steps, you'll gradually integrate the principles of the East Asian diet into your daily routine. Remember, it's about making mindful choices that honor the balance between taste and nutrition. Enjoy the journey of discovering new foods and flavors that contribute to a healthier, more balanced lifestyle.

Foods Included in the East Asian Diet Plan

The East Asian Diet is varied, with cuisines spanning numerous countries including China, Japan, the Korean countries, Taiwan, Vietnam, Thailand, Malaysia, Indonesia, the Philippines, Cambodia, and other countries.

While the spices and the way of cooking vary from country to country, what is constant is that these regional diets are connected with the use of organic, fresh, and natural foods. The East Asian Diet includes vegetables, grains, fruits, and meat.

- *Vegetables*. These include cabbage, broccoli, lettuce, celery, bok choy, kale, and spinach. Non-leafy vegetables include cauliflower, carrots, turnips, eggplant, green peppers, and radishes. Some Asian supermarkets also carry vegetables like lotus root, bamboo, Chinese yam, and winter melon.
- *Meat*. Meat is consumed in moderation in the East Asian Diet. Some acceptable meats include lean meat like duck, fish, chicken, and pork. Beef is not always consumed. In place of meat, vegetarians eat eggs, while vegan consume tofu.
- *Fruit*. The East Asian Diet includes fruits like oranges, apples, grapes, bananas, mangoes, pears, pineapple, strawberries, and watermelon.
- *Grains*. Rice is a staple in the East Asian Diet. However, rice has numerous varieties like short-grain, long-grain, white rice, jasmine rice, brown rice, red rice, millet, purple rice, and black rice. Wheat is eaten in the form of steamed buns, bread, and noodles.

Foods to Avoid

When adopting an East Asian diet, which is renowned for its focus on whole, plant-based foods and minimal consumption of meat and dairy, there are certain foods you might consider avoiding or consuming with caution to maximize health benefits. Based on the context provided, here's a list of foods to be mindful of:

1. ***Fish and Shellfish***: While an essential part of the diet for their omega-3 fatty acids and protein, some may be high in mercury or other contaminants. It's advisable to choose low-mercury options and ensure proper preparation.
2. ***Fried Rice***: A common dish that can be high in calories and unhealthy fats due to the cooking process. Opting for brown rice or steamed versions could be healthier.
3. ***Raw Eggs***: Used in various dishes, raw eggs carry a risk of salmonella. It's important to use fresh eggs and consider the potential risks, especially for vulnerable populations.
4. ***Undercooked Meat***: Consuming undercooked meat increases the risk of foodborne illnesses. Ensure meats are cooked to safe internal temperatures.
5. ***Salad or Raw Vegetables***: In areas where water sanitation is a concern, consuming raw vegetables may increase exposure to contaminants. Washing

thoroughly or opting for cooked vegetables can mitigate this risk.

6. ***High-Sodium Foods***: Many sauces, like soy sauce, used in East Asian cooking are high in sodium, which can impact blood pressure and heart health. Seeking low-sodium alternatives or using them sparingly is beneficial.
7. ***Instant Noodles***: Although convenient, they're often high in sodium and trans fats, offering little nutritional value. Limiting consumption and choosing whole-grain options when possible is recommended.
8. ***Sugary Foods and Beverages***: Traditional desserts and sweetened beverages can contribute to excessive sugar intake. Moderation is key, as is opting for fruits or unsweetened alternatives for a sweet fix.
9. ***Barbecue Spare Ribs***: A popular but high-fat choice, often coated in salty-sweet sauces. Opting for leaner meats and reducing sauce intake can help balance the meal.

By being mindful of these foods within the context of the East Asian diet, individuals can enjoy the myriad health benefits this dietary approach offers while minimizing potential risks.

Sample 7-Day Meal Plan

The East Asian Diet is different from the typical American and Western diets in the sense that the former is a simple activity. There is no need to think about the order of consuming food from soup to salad to the main course to dessert. Snacking in the East Asian Diet is not complicated. Sometimes, all you need to eat for snacks can just be a few pieces of dried fruit, nuts, or a combination of both.

The East Asian Diet works to promote wellness and weight loss in several ways. Below are some reasons why the East Asian Diet is better than the average Western diet when it comes to weight loss.

- ***Organic, Natural, and Fresh***. Many East Asian recipes call for organic, natural, and fresh ingredients. Processed, artificial, or frozen ingredients are rarely used.
- ***Low-Calorie, Yet Flavorful***. Since the East Asian Diet is comprised mostly of vegetables, the recipes belonging to the diet have a low-calorie count. You can afford to eat in large quantities and not gain weight.

East Asian dishes are also flavorful. Thus, attaining wellness with this diet is an enjoyable adventure.

- *Manageable Portions*. The East Asian Diet calls for small plates and bowls, which is vital for weight loss as it allows you to easily manage portions. Eat the food in your bowl, and you won't have to worry about overeating.
- *Metabolism and Digestion are Important*. Good digestion raises your metabolism. Asian people normally eat hot food. They also avoid cold drinks and food with their meals. Vegetable dishes are also rich in fiber. Eating a lot of meat also lowers metabolism, which is the reason why Asians eat meat moderately.

Below is a sample seven-day meal plan to highlight the simplicity of the East Asian Diet.

Day 1

Breakfast: Roasted Chicken Banh Mi

Lunch: Chicken Thigh Hoisin-Style with Salad

Dinner: Miso Vegetable Soup

Day 2

Breakfast: Shrimp Fried Rice

Lunch: Ginger Beef Stir-Fry with Bok Choy

Dinner: Spinach Salad Mixed with Ginger Dressing

Day 3

Breakfast: Kimchi Fried Rice

Lunch: Cantonese-Style Vegetable and Chicken Combo

Dinner: Chinese Noodle Salad with Sesame Dressing

Day 4

Breakfast: Peanut Butter Noodles

Lunch: Cantonese Shiu Mai

Dinner: Spinach Seasoned Korean Style

Day 5

Breakfast: Fresh Spring Rolls

Lunch: Broccoli with Cashews and Garlic Butter

Dinner: Korean Bean Sprout Salad

Day 6

Breakfast: Fish Congee

Lunch: Chicken Soba Noodles

Dinner: Egg Fried Rice

Day 7

Breakfast: Rice Congee

Lunch: Hot Noodle Soup

Dinner: Chicken & Green Pepper Stir Fry

Sample Recipes

We've talked about the principles of the East Asian diet and its health benefits, but it's always helpful to see some sample recipes in action. Here are a few delicious and simple dishes to try out at home!

Roasted Chicken Banh Mi

Ingredients:

For the Chicken:

- 2 boneless, skinless chicken breasts
- 2 cloves garlic, minced
- 1 tablespoon low-sodium soy sauce
- 1 tablespoon fish sauce
- 1 teaspoon honey
- 1/2 teaspoon freshly ground black pepper

For the Pickled Vegetables:

- 1/2 cup distilled white vinegar
- 1 tablespoon sugar
- 1 teaspoon salt
- 1 carrot, julienned
- 1 daikon radish, julienned

For the Sandwich:

- 4 whole-grain baguettes or sandwich rolls, split open
- Light mayonnaise (optional)
- Fresh cilantro leaves
- Thinly sliced cucumber
- Thinly sliced jalapeño (optional, for heat)
- Low-sodium soy sauce, to taste

Instructions:

1. In a bowl, combine garlic, low-sodium soy sauce, fish sauce, honey, and black pepper. Add the chicken breasts, ensuring they are well-coated with the marinade. Cover and refrigerate for at least 1 hour, or overnight for more flavor.
2. In another bowl, whisk together white vinegar, sugar, and salt until dissolved. Add the julienned carrot and daikon radish. Let sit for at least 30 minutes, stirring occasionally.
3. Preheat your oven to 375°F (190°C). Place the marinated chicken breasts on a baking sheet and roast for 25-30 minutes, or until the chicken is thoroughly cooked and juices run clear. Once done, let the chicken rest for a few minutes, then slice thinly.
4. Lightly toast the whole-grain baguettes or rolls. Spread a thin layer of light mayonnaise on each side of the bread (optional). Arrange slices of roasted chicken on the bread.
5. Drain the pickled vegetables and add them generously on top of the chicken. Add slices of cucumber and jalapeño (if using) for an extra crunch and kick.
6. Garnish with fresh cilantro leaves. Drizzle a bit of low-sodium soy sauce over the filling for an added depth of flavor.
7. Close the sandwiches, cut in half, and serve immediately.

Chicken Thigh Hoisin-Style with Salad

Ingredients:

For the Chicken:

- 4 boneless, skinless chicken thighs
- 2 tablespoons hoisin sauce (ensure it's low sodium)
- 1 tablespoon honey (or a substitute like agave syrup for a lower glycemic index)
- 1 tablespoon soy sauce (low sodium)
- 2 cloves garlic, minced
- 1 teaspoon grated fresh ginger
- 1 teaspoon sesame oil
- Optional: A pinch of Chinese Five Spice for added flavor

For the Salad:

- 2 cups mixed greens (spinach, kale, arugula)
- 1 small carrot, julienned
- 1/2 cucumber, thinly sliced
- 1/4 red bell pepper, thinly sliced
- 1 tablespoon rice vinegar
- 1 teaspoon sesame seeds

Instructions:

Prepare the Chicken:

1. Marinate: In a large bowl, whisk together the hoisin sauce, honey, soy sauce, garlic, ginger, and sesame oil. Add the chicken thighs, ensuring they are fully coated with the marinade. Cover and let marinate in the refrigerator for at least 1 hour, or overnight for more depth of flavor.
2. Cook: Preheat your oven to 375°F (190°C). Place the marinated chicken thighs on a baking tray lined with parchment paper. Bake for 25-30 minutes, or until the chicken is cooked through and the outside is caramelized. Optionally, you can finish the chicken under the broiler for 2-3 minutes for extra crispiness.
3. Combine Vegetables: In a large salad bowl, mix the mixed greens, carrot, cucumber, and red bell pepper.
4. Dressing: Drizzle the rice vinegar over the salad and toss to coat evenly. Sprinkle sesame seeds on top for a crunchy finish.
5. Slice the cooked chicken thighs and place them atop the prepared salad. Serve immediately while the chicken is warm.

Miso Vegetable Soup Recipe

Ingredients:

- 4 cups vegetable broth (low sodium preferred)
- 2-3 tablespoons miso paste (ensure it's organic and non-GMO for best quality)
- 1 sheet nori seaweed, torn into pieces
- 1/2 cup tofu, cubed (soft or silken for traditional texture)
- 1 cup mushrooms, thinly sliced (shiitake or button mushrooms work well)
- 1 small carrot, julienned
- 1 small daikon radish, julienned (optional for added crunch and flavor)
- 2 green onions, chopped
- 1/2 cup baby spinach or kale leaves
- 1 teaspoon sesame oil (for flavor, optional)

Instructions:

1. Prepare the Broth: In a large pot, bring the vegetable broth to a simmer over medium heat.
2. Dissolve the Miso: In a small bowl, mix the miso paste with a little hot water from the pot until it becomes a smooth liquid. This prevents clumps of miso in your soup. Set aside.
3. Add the Vegetables: To the simmering broth, add the tofu, mushrooms, carrot, and daikon radish. Let them

simmer gently for about 5 minutes, or until they start to soften.
4. Incorporate Miso: Reduce the heat to low, and carefully stir in the dissolved miso paste to the pot. It's important not to let the soup boil after adding miso to preserve its flavor and health benefits.
5. Final Touches: Add the torn nori seaweed, green onions, and leafy greens (spinach or kale). Simmer on low heat for another 2-3 minutes, just until the greens wilt and the flavors meld together.
6. Serve: Drizzle with a teaspoon of sesame oil for an added depth of flavor (optional). Serve the soup warm in bowls, ensuring that there are equal portions of the vegetables and tofu in each.

Shrimp Fried Rice

Ingredients:

- 1 cup brown rice (or a mix of brown and wild rice for added texture and nutrients)
- 2 cups water (for cooking rice)
- 1 tablespoon coconut oil or olive oil
- 2 cloves garlic, minced
- 1-inch piece of ginger, minced
- 1/2 pound (about 225 grams) shrimp, peeled and deveined
- 1 cup mixed vegetables (carrots, peas, bell peppers), finely chopped
- 2 green onions, thinly sliced
- 1 egg, lightly beaten (optional)
- 2 tablespoons low-sodium soy sauce or tamari
- 1 teaspoon sesame oil
- Freshly ground black pepper, to taste

Instructions:

1. Prepare Rice: Rinse the brown rice under cold water until the water runs clear. In a pot, bring 2 cups of water to a boil. Add the rice, reduce heat to low, cover, and simmer for 45 minutes or until the rice is cooked and water is absorbed. Let it cool, preferably refrigerate for a few hours or overnight for best results.

2. Sauté Aromatics: In a large skillet or wok, heat the coconut or olive oil over medium-high heat. Add the minced garlic and ginger, sautéing for about 1 minute until fragrant.
3. Cook Shrimp: Add the shrimp to the skillet and cook until they turn pink and opaque, about 2-3 minutes per side. Remove the shrimp from the skillet and set aside.
4. Vegetables: In the same skillet, add the chopped mixed vegetables and cook until they're tender but still crisp about 3-5 minutes.
5. Combine: Push the vegetables to one side of the skillet. If using an egg, pour the beaten egg into the other side of the skillet and scramble until fully cooked. Then, mix the scrambled egg with the vegetables.
6. Season: Drizzle low-sodium soy sauce, and sesame oil, and sprinkle freshly ground black pepper over the rice mixture. Stir well to combine all the ingredients and ensure the rice is heated through.
7. Final Touches: Add the sliced green onions, give the mixture a final stir, and remove from heat.

Ginger Beef Stir-Fry with Bok Choy

Ingredients:

- 1 pound beef (450g) flank steak, thinly sliced against the grain
- 2 tablespoons soy sauce (or tamari for a gluten-free option)
- 1 tablespoon fresh ginger, grated
- 1 garlic clove, minced
- 1 teaspoon sesame oil
- 2 cups bok choy, washed and chopped
- 1 red bell pepper, thinly sliced
- 1 carrot, julienned
- 1 onion, thinly sliced
- 1/4 cup low-sodium chicken broth or water
- 1 tablespoon oyster sauce
- 1 teaspoon cornstarch (optional, for thickening)
- 1 tablespoon soy sauce
- 1 teaspoon sesame oil
- 1 teaspoon honey (optional, adjust based on dietary restrictions)
- 2 tablespoons vegetable oil, divided
- Sesame seeds
- Green onions, thinly sliced

Instructions:

1. Marinade Preparation: Mix soy sauce, ginger, garlic, and sesame oil in a bowl. Coat thinly sliced beef in the marinade and let it marinate for at least 15 minutes, or up to an hour in the fridge for more flavor.
2. Sauce Preparation: Whisk chicken broth, oyster sauce, soy sauce, sesame oil, cornstarch (optional), and honey (optional) in a small bowl. Set aside.
3. Beef Stir-Fry: Heat 1 tablespoon of vegetable oil in a large pan or wok over high heat. Cook marinated beef in batches until browned evenly, about 2 minutes per side. Remove from pan.
4. Vegetables: Add more oil if needed. Stir-fry onion, bell pepper, and carrot for 3-4 minutes until soft. Add bok choy and stir-fry for 2 minutes until wilted.
5. Combining: Mix beef, vegetables, and sauce in the pan. Cook for 1-2 minutes to thicken the sauce.
6. Serving: Enjoy the Ginger Beef Stir-Fry hot, topped with sesame seeds and green onions if desired. Goes well with rice or noodles.

Spinach Salad Mixed with Ginger Dressing

Ingredients:

- 4 cups fresh spinach leaves, washed and dried
- 1 cup shredded carrots
- 1/2 cup sliced cucumber
- 1/4 cup thinly sliced red onion
- 1/4 cup edamame (shelled)
- 1 tablespoon toasted sesame seeds
- 2 tablespoons soy sauce (or tamari for a gluten-free option)
- 1 tablespoon rice vinegar
- 1 tablespoon freshly grated ginger
- 1 teaspoon sesame oil
- 1 teaspoon honey (optional, can adjust or omit based on dietary needs)
- 1 clove garlic, minced
- 1 teaspoon finely chopped green onion

Instructions:

1. Prepare Salad: Mix spinach leaves, shredded carrots, cucumber, red onion, and edamame in a large bowl. Toss gently.
2. Make Ginger Dressing: Whisk soy sauce, rice vinegar, grated ginger, sesame oil, honey (optional), garlic, and green onion in a small bowl until combined. Adjust seasoning to taste.

3. Combine & Serve: Pour ginger dressing over the salad, and toss gently to coat evenly.
4. Sprinkle toasted sesame seeds for crunch and flavor.
5. Serve Immediately: Enjoy fresh. Serve right after dressing for the best texture and flavor.

Cantonese-Style Vegetable and Chicken Combo

Ingredients:

- 1 pound (450g) chicken breast, cut into bite-size pieces
- 1 tablespoon low-sodium soy sauce (or tamari for gluten-free)
- 1 teaspoon cornstarch
- 1/2 cup red bell pepper, sliced
- 1/2 cup green beans, trimmed
- 1/2 cup baby corn, halved lengthwise
- 1/2 cup broccoli florets
- 1/4 cup carrots, julienned
- 2 tablespoons water chestnuts, sliced (optional)
- 1 cup low-sodium chicken broth or water
- 1 tablespoon oyster sauce
- 1 teaspoon soy sauce
- 1 teaspoon sesame oil
- 1/2 teaspoon honey (optional, adjust based on dietary restrictions)
- 1 teaspoon cornstarch (dissolved in 2 tablespoons water for thickening)
- 2 tablespoons vegetable oil, divided
- 2 cloves garlic, minced
- 1 tablespoon fresh ginger, minced

Instructions:

1. Marinate the Chicken: Mix chicken with 1 tbsp soy sauce and 1 tsp cornstarch. Let marinate for 15 minutes.
2. Prepare the Sauce: Whisk chicken broth, oyster sauce, soy sauce, sesame oil, and honey (optional) with dissolved cornstarch. Set aside.
3. Cook the Chicken: Heat 1 tbsp vegetable oil in a pan. Stir-fry chicken until cooked, about 5-6 minutes. Remove and set aside.
4. Stir-Fry the Vegetables: In the same pan, add 1 tbsp vegetable oil. Cook garlic, ginger, and vegetables for 3-4 minutes.
5. Combine Chicken and Vegetables: Return chicken to the pan with vegetables. Pour sauce over and mix well. Cook for 2-3 minutes until sauce thickens.
6. Serve: Enjoy the Cantonese-style vegetable and Chicken Combo hot with steamed jasmine or brown rice.

Kimchi Fried Rice

Ingredients:

- 2 cups cooked rice (preferably day-old rice as it fries better)
- 1 cup well-fermented kimchi, chopped
- 1/4 cup kimchi juice (for flavor and color)
- 2 tablespoons vegetable oil
- 1 tablespoon sesame oil
- 1 tablespoon soy sauce (or tamari for a gluten-free option)
- 1 teaspoon gochujang (Korean chili paste, adjust according to spice preference)
- 2 green onions, chopped
- 1 clove garlic, minced
- 1/2 onion, finely diced
- 1/2 cup mixed vegetables (such as carrots, peas, and corn) - use fresh or frozen
- Optional for serving: roasted seaweed strips, toasted sesame seeds, fried egg (omit for vegan)

Instructions:

1. Prepare Ingredients: Ensure cooked and chilled rice. This prevents mushiness when frying. Chop kimchi into bite-sized pieces.
2. Cook Aromatics: Heat oil in skillet. Sauté garlic and onion until soft and fragrant, about 2 minutes.

3. Add Kimchi: Stir in kimchi and cook for 2 minutes until slightly caramelized.
4. Mix Rice and Seasonings: Add rice, kimchi juice, soy sauce, and gochujang. Stir to combine. Cook until slightly crispy, about 5 minutes.
5. Add Vegetables: Mix in vegetables and cook until tender, 3-4 minutes.
6. Final Touches: Drizzle sesame oil, add green onions, leaving some for garnish.
7. Serve: Hot, garnished with remaining green onions, sesame seeds, and roasted seaweed strips. Top with a fried egg for extra protein (optional).

Chinese Noodle Salad with Sesame Dressing

Ingredients:

- 8 ounces whole wheat noodles or soba noodles
- 1 cup shredded purple cabbage
- 1/2 cup shredded carrots
- 1/2 cup thinly sliced cucumber
- 1/4 cup thinly sliced green onions
- 1/4 cup chopped cilantro (optional)
- 1 tablespoon sesame seeds (for garnish)
- 3 tablespoons low-sodium soy sauce (or tamari for gluten-free)
- 2 tablespoons rice vinegar
- 1 tablespoon toasted sesame oil
- 1 teaspoon honey (adjust according to taste; can be omitted)
- 1 tablespoon natural peanut butter or tahini
- 1 clove garlic, minced
- 1 teaspoon grated fresh ginger

Instructions:

1. Cook the Noodles: Cook noodles per package instructions until al dente. Rinse under cold water, drain well, and set aside.
2. Prepare the Vegetables: While noodles cook, prep cabbage, carrots, cucumber, green onions, and cilantro. Set aside.

3. Make the Sesame Dressing: In a small bowl, whisk soy sauce, rice vinegar, toasted sesame oil, honey (if using), peanut butter or tahini, garlic, and ginger until smooth.
4. Combine Salad and Dressing: In a large bowl, mix cooked noodles, veggies, and cilantro (if using). Pour dressing over and toss to coat.
5. Garnish and Serve: Transfer salad to a dish, and sprinkle sesame seeds as garnish. Serve chilled or at room temperature.

Peanut Butter Noodles

Ingredients:

- 8 ounces of your preferred noodles (whole wheat spaghetti, soba, or rice noodles for gluten-free options)
- 1/3 cup natural peanut butter (unsweetened and unsalted)
- 1/4 cup low-sodium soy sauce or tamari (for gluten-free)
- 2 tablespoons rice vinegar
- 1 tablespoon toasted sesame oil
- 1 teaspoon minced fresh ginger
- 2 cloves garlic, minced
- 1-2 teaspoons chili paste or chili oil (adjust to taste)
- 1 tablespoon honey or maple syrup (optional, adjust based on dietary needs)
- Hot water (as needed to thin the sauce)
- For garnish: chopped green onions, sesame seeds, and/or crushed peanuts

Instructions:

1. Cook the Noodles: Follow package instructions to cook noodles until al dente. Drain, rinse with cold water, and set aside.
2. Prepare the Peanut Sauce: In a bowl, mix natural peanut butter, low-sodium soy sauce, rice vinegar, toasted sesame oil, minced ginger, minced garlic, chili

paste, and honey or maple syrup. Whisk until smooth. Add hot water gradually if needed for consistency.
3. Combine Noodles and Sauce: Toss cooked noodles with peanut sauce until coated evenly. Add hot water if dry.
4. Serve: Garnish noodles with green onions, sesame seeds, and crushed peanuts. Enjoy warm or chilled for any occasion.

Korean-Style Seasoned Spinach (Sigeumchi Namul)

Ingredients:

- 1 lb (450g) fresh spinach
- 2 cloves garlic, minced
- 2 green onions, finely chopped
- 1 tablespoon low-sodium soy sauce
- 1 tablespoon sesame oil
- 1 teaspoon sesame seeds
- Salt to taste
- A pinch of sugar or natural sweetener (optional)

Instructions:

1. Wash the spinach thoroughly. Blanch in boiling water with a pinch of salt for 30 seconds to 1 minute, then plunge into ice water. Drain and squeeze out excess water.
2. In a bowl, mix the spinach with garlic, green onions, soy sauce, sesame oil, and a pinch of sugar or sweetener if using.
3. Adjust seasoning to taste. Transfer to a serving dish and sprinkle with sesame seeds.
4. Serve immediately or chilled.

Fresh Spring Rolls with Peanut Dipping Sauce

Ingredients:

- 8 spring roll wrappers (rice paper)
- 1 cup cooked vermicelli noodles
- 1 carrot, julienned or grated
- 1 cucumber, julienned or thinly sliced
- 1 avocado, thinly sliced
- 1/2 red bell pepper, thinly sliced
- 1/4 cup fresh cilantro, chopped
- 1/4 cup fresh mint leaves

Peanut Dipping Sauce:

- 1/3 cup creamy peanut butter
- 2 tablespoons low-sodium soy sauce
- 2 tablespoons rice vinegar
- 2 teaspoons honey or natural sweetener
- 1 clove garlic, minced
- 1 teaspoon grated ginger
- Water, as needed for thinning out sauce

Instructions:

1. In a large bowl of warm water, soak one spring roll wrapper at a time for about 10 seconds until softened.
2. Transfer the wrapper to a flat surface and place desired fillings in the center, leaving some space on either side.

3. Start with a small amount of each filling and add more as needed to avoid overfilling the wrapper.
4. Roll up the bottom edge of the wrapper over the fillings, then fold in both sides towards the center. Continue rolling tightly until sealed.
5. Repeat with remaining spring roll wrappers and fillings.
6. To make the peanut dipping sauce, mix all ingredients in a small bowl until smooth. Add water as needed to thin out the sauce to the desired consistency.
7. Serve spring rolls with peanut dipping sauce on the side for dipping. Enjoy!

Mixed Berry Smoothie Bowl

Ingredients:

- 1 cup frozen mixed berries
- 1 banana, sliced and frozen
- 1/2 cup plain Greek yogurt
- 1/4 cup almond milk
- Toppings of choice (granola, fresh berries, nuts, etc.)

Instructions:

1. In a blender, combine frozen berries, frozen banana, Greek yogurt, and almond milk. Blend until smooth.
2. Pour mixture into a bowl.
3. Add desired toppings such as granola, fresh berries, or nuts.
4. Enjoy your delicious and nutritious mixed berry smoothie bowl!

Broccoli with Cashews and Garlic Butter

Ingredients:

- 1 head of broccoli, cut into florets
- 2 tablespoons olive oil
- 3 cloves of garlic, minced
- 1/4 cup cashews, roughly chopped
- Salt and pepper, to taste

Instructions:

1. In a large skillet, heat olive oil over medium-high heat.
2. Add broccoli florets and cook for 5-7 minutes, stirring occasionally until tender.
3. Add minced garlic to the skillet and continue cooking for an additional 1-2 minutes until fragrant.
4. Season with salt and pepper to taste.
5. In a separate small pan, toast chopped cashews over medium heat for about 3 minutes until lightly browned.
6. Add toasted cashews to the skillet with broccoli and garlic.
7. Toss everything together and let cook for an additional 1-2 minutes.
8. Serve hot as a side dish or over rice for a complete meal. Enjoy!

Fish Congee

Ingredients:

- 1 cup jasmine rice
- 4 cups chicken or vegetable broth
- 2 cups water
- 1 pound white fish fillets, such as cod or tilapia, cut into bite-sized pieces
- 1-inch piece of ginger, peeled and minced
- 3 cloves of garlic, minced
- Salt and pepper, to taste
- Optional toppings: sliced green onions, cilantro, sesame oil, soy sauce

Instructions:

1. In a large pot, bring the chicken or vegetable broth and water to a boil.
2. Rinse the jasmine rice in cold water until the water runs clear. Add it to the boiling broth and reduce heat to medium-low.
3. Let the rice cook for 15 minutes, stirring occasionally to prevent sticking.
4. Add the minced ginger and garlic to the pot and let it cook for an additional 5 minutes.
5. Season with salt and pepper to taste.
6. Gently add in the fish fillets, making sure they are fully submerged in the broth.

7. Let everything simmer for about 10 minutes until the fish is fully cooked and the congee has reached a creamy consistency.
8. Serve hot and garnish with your desired toppings, such as sliced green onions, cilantro, sesame oil, or soy sauce. Enjoy this comforting and nourishing dish!

Chicken & Green Pepper Stir Fry

Ingredients:

- 1 pound boneless, skinless chicken breast or thighs, cut into bite-sized pieces
- 2 tablespoons cornstarch
- Salt and pepper, to taste
- 2 tablespoons vegetable oil
- 1 green bell pepper, seeded and sliced
- 1 onion, sliced
- 2 cloves of garlic, minced
- 1/4 cup chicken broth
- 2 tablespoons soy sauce

Instructions:

1. In a small bowl, mix together the chicken pieces, cornstarch, salt and pepper until the chicken is evenly coated.
2. Heat the vegetable oil in a large skillet over medium-high heat.
3. Add the chicken to the skillet and cook for 5-6 minutes, stirring occasionally, until it is fully cooked.
4. Remove the chicken from the skillet and set aside on a plate.
5. In the same skillet, add in the sliced green bell peppers, onion, and minced garlic. Cook for 3-4 minutes until they are slightly softened.

6. Pour in the chicken broth and soy sauce, and stir to combine with the vegetables.
7. Let the mixture cook for an additional 2-3 minutes until the sauce has thickened and coats the vegetables.
8. Add the cooked chicken back into the skillet and toss everything together to evenly coat with the sauce.
9. Serve hot over rice or noodles for a deliciously simple dinner option. You can also add in other vegetables like carrots, mushrooms, or broccoli for added nutrition and flavor. Enjoy this tasty and easy stir-fry dish!

Cantonese Shiu Mai Dumplings

Ingredients:

- 1/2 pound ground pork
- 1/4 cup chopped shrimp
- 1/4 cup grated carrot
- 1 green onion, finely chopped
- 2 cloves of garlic, minced
- 1 tablespoon soy sauce
- 1 teaspoon sesame oil
- Wonton wrappers

Instructions:

1. In a mixing bowl, combine the ground pork, chopped shrimp, grated carrot, green onion, minced garlic, soy sauce, and sesame oil.
2. Mix all of the ingredients together until well combined.
3. Place a wonton wrapper on a flat surface and spoon approximately 1 tablespoon of the mixture into the center of the wrapper.
4. Wet the edges of the wrapper with water and fold it into a small parcel, pinching the edges together to seal.
5. Repeat until all of the mixture has been used up.
6. Heat a large pot of water over high heat and bring to a boil.

7. Place the dumplings in the boiling water and let them cook for 6-8 minutes until they float to the surface and are fully cooked.
8. Remove the dumplings from the water with a slotted spoon and let them drain on a paper towel-lined plate.
9. Serve hot with soy sauce or your favorite dipping sauce. You can also steam these dumplings for 10-12 minutes instead of boiling them for a healthier option. Enjoy this classic Cantonese dish as a delicious appetizer or main course meal!

Conclusion

As you reach the conclusion of our East Asian diet guide, take a moment to reflect on the journey you've embarked upon. By exploring the rich tapestry of flavors, ingredients, and culinary traditions that define East Asian cuisine, you've not only broadened your palate but also taken meaningful steps towards embracing a lifestyle that champions balance, health, and wellness. Your commitment to understanding and integrating these dietary principles into your life is commendable, and it's an accomplishment worth celebrating.

The East Asian diet, renowned for its emphasis on whole, minimally processed foods, stands as a testament to the wisdom of traditional eating habits that have been cultivated over millennia. The incorporation of a wide variety of vegetables, whole grains, lean proteins, and healthy fats, complemented by cooking methods that preserve the natural goodness of these ingredients, exemplifies a diet that nourishes the body and soul. This approach to eating not only supports physical health but also fosters a deeper connection with food, encouraging mindful eating practices that enhance our overall well-being.

Throughout this guide, you've been introduced to the core components of the East Asian diet and discovered how these elements work in harmony to promote longevity and vitality. The sample recipes provided have offered a glimpse into the art of East Asian cooking, showcasing how simple, yet flavorful, dishes can be crafted from basic ingredients. From the heartwarming comfort of a bowl of congee to the refreshing crispness of a cucumber salad, each recipe serves as a building block for a diet that is as nutritious as it is satisfying.

As you move forward, armed with new knowledge and culinary skills, remember that the journey to embracing the East Asian diet is a personal one, shaped by individual tastes, preferences, and lifestyle considerations. There's no one-size-fits-all approach, and the beauty of this diet lies in its flexibility and adaptability. Experiment with different ingredients, explore new flavors and don't hesitate to modify recipes to suit your needs. The goal is to find joy and fulfillment in the meals you prepare, creating a sustainable eating pattern that resonates with you.

Thank you for taking the time to delve into the East Asian diet with us. Your dedication to exploring new culinary horizons and prioritizing your health is inspiring. As you continue on this path, be encouraged by the progress you've made and the discoveries you've yet to make. Remember, every meal is an opportunity to nourish your body, celebrate cultural traditions, and cultivate a sense of well-being that extends beyond the dinner table.

So, here's to your journey—a journey filled with delicious discoveries, healthful choices, and endless possibilities. Keep exploring, keep experimenting, and most importantly, keep enjoying every bite. Your adventure in the world of East Asian cuisine has only just begun, and we can't wait to see where it takes you. Here's to your health, happiness, and a future brimming with flavorful, nourishing meals. Cheers to you and your continued success on this culinary journey!

FAQ

What is the East Asian Diet?

The East Asian Diet is a way of eating based on the traditional dietary patterns of countries like China, Japan, and Korea. It focuses on whole, plant-based foods including a variety of produce, legumes, whole grains, lean proteins (especially fish), and minimally processed foods.

What are the key components of the East Asian Diet?

Key components include a high intake of vegetables and fruits, whole grains, soy products such as tofu and soy sauce, seafood, and a moderate consumption of poultry and eggs. Red meat is eaten sparingly, and meals are often flavored with herbs and spices instead of heavy sauces or salts.

How does the East Asian Diet differ from Western diets?

The East Asian Diet places a greater emphasis on plant-based foods and fish, which contributes to a lower intake of saturated fats and processed foods. It also prioritizes rice and noodles as staple carbohydrates over bread and pasta and favors tea over sugary drinks.

Can the East Asian Diet aid in weight management?

Yes, due to its focus on whole, nutrient-dense foods and lower consumption of processed foods and unhealthy fats, the East Asian Diet can help in maintaining a healthy weight. Portion control and the balance of food groups also play a crucial role in its effectiveness for weight management.

What are some health benefits associated with the East Asian Diet?

Adhering to the East Asian Diet can lead to numerous health benefits, including improved cardiovascular health, better digestion, reduced risk of chronic diseases such as diabetes and certain cancers, and enhanced overall well-being.

Are there any cultural aspects to consider when adopting the East Asian Diet?

Yes, the East Asian Diet is not just about food choices but also involves cultural practices such as mindful eating, appreciating the flavors and textures of food, and sharing meals with family or friends. Understanding and respecting these cultural elements can enrich the experience of adopting this diet.

How can someone get started with the East Asian Diet?

Getting started involves incorporating more vegetables, fruits, and whole grains into your meals, choosing fish and plant-based proteins, and reducing the intake of processed foods and red meats. Experimenting with traditional East Asian recipes and flavors can also help ease the transition and make the diet more enjoyable.

References and Helpful Links

Bedosky, L. (2022, July 28). What is the Asian diet? potential health benefits, food list, meal plan, and more. EverydayHealth.com. https://www.everydayhealth.com/diet-nutrition/what-is-the-asian-diet-potential-health-benefits-food-list-meal-plan-and-more/#:~:text=What%20is%20the%20typical%20Asian,with%20minimal%20meat%20and%20dairy

Eating well with Diabetes: East Asian diets - Unlock Food. (n.d.). https://www.unlockfood.ca/en/Articles/Diabetes/Diabetes-and-Healthy-Eating/Eating-well-with-Diabetes-East-Asian-diets.aspx

Admin. (2024, February 19). What is the Asian Diet for Weight Loss? United Bariatric Center of Kansas City. https://kc-weightloss.com/asian-diet-weight-loss/

Om, C. M. L. D. (2014, January 23). 10 things you need to know about the Asian diet. HuffPost. https://www.huffpost.com/entry/asian-diet_b_4015133

Healthy Asian meal plan to lose weight (Breakfast, lunch, dinner). (n.d.). http://www.joannasoh.com/foods/recipes-1/healthy-asian-meal-plan-to-lose-weight-breakfast-lunch-dinner

Lindberg, S., & OksanaKiian/iStock/GettyImages. (2019, December 5). Asian meal plans to lose weight in 7 days. Livestrong.com.

https://www.livestrong.com/article/318146-asian-meal-plans-to-lose-weight-in-7-days/

East Asian recipes. (2021, March 23). Serious Eats. https://www.seriouseats.com/east-asian-recipes-5117260

www.ingramcontent.com/pod-product-compliance
Lightning Source LLC
LaVergne TN
LVHW021229080526
838199LV00089B/5960